Spirituality in Nursing

Spirituality in Nursing

AM Rajinikanth
MSc N PhD (Psy)
Lecturer
Vidyakirana Institute of Nursing Sciences
Bangalore 560 076

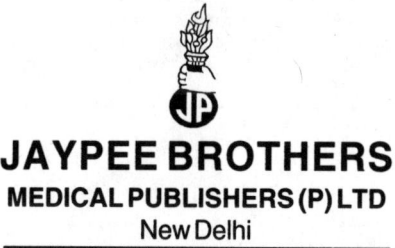

JAYPEE BROTHERS
MEDICAL PUBLISHERS (P) LTD
New Delhi

Published by
Jitendar P Vij
Jaypee Brothers Medical Publishers (P) Ltd
EMCA House, 23/23B Ansari Road, Daryaganj
New Delhi 110 002, India Phones: +91-11-23272143, +91-11-23272703,
+91-11-23282021, +91-11-23245672 Fax: +91-11-23276490, +91-11-23245683
e-mail: jaypee@jaypeebrothers.com
Visit our website: www.jaypeebrothers.com

Branches

- 2/B, Akruti Society, Jodhpur Gam Road Satellite, **Ahmedabad** 380 015
  Phones: +91-079-30988717, +91-079-26926233   e-mail: jpamdvd@rediffmail.com
- 202 Batavia Chambers, 8 Kumara Krupa Road
  Kumara Park East, **Bangalore** 560 001
  Phones: +91-80-22285971, +91-80-22382956, +91-80-30614073
  Tele Fax: +91-80-22281761   e-mail: jaypeemedpubbgl@eth.net
- 282 IIIrd Floor, Khaleel Shirazi Estate, Fountain Plaza
  Pantheon Road, **Chennai** 600 008
  Phones: +91-44-28193265, +91-44-28194897
  Fax: +91-44-28193231   e-mail: jpchen@eth.net
- 4-2-1067/1-3, Ist Floor, Balaji Building, Ramkote, Cross Road, **Hyderabad** 500 095
  Phones: +91-40-55610020, +91-40-24758498, +91-40-30940929
  Fax: +91-40-24758499   e-mail: jpmedpub@rediffmail.com
- 1A Indian Mirror Street, Wellington Square, **Kolkata** 700 013
  Phones: +91-33-22456075 , +91-33-22451926 , +91-33-30901926
  Fax: +91-33-22456075   e-mail: jpbcal@cal.vsnl.net.in
- 106 Amit Industrial Estate, 61 Dr SS Rao Road
  Near MGM Hospital Parel, **Mumbai** 400 012
  Phones: +91-22-24124863, +91-22-24104532, +91-22-30926896
  Fax: +91-22-24160828   e-mail: jpmedpub@bom7.vsnl.net.in
- "KAMALPUSHPA" 38, Reshimbag, Opp. Mohota Science College,
  Umred Road, **Nagpur** 440 009, Phones: +91-712-3945220, +91-712-2704275
  Fax: 0712-2704275   e-mail: jpmednagpur@rediffmail.com

Spirituality in Nursing

© 2006, AM Rajinikanth

All rights reserved. No part of this publication should be reproduced, stored in a retrieval system, or transmitted in any form or by any means: electronic, mechanical, photocopying, recording, or otherwise, without the prior written permission of the author and the publisher.

> This book has been published in good faith that the material provided by author is original. Every effort is made to ensure accuracy of material, but the publisher, printer and author will not be held responsible for any inadvertent error(s). In case of any dispute, all legal matters are to be settled under Delhi jurisdiction only.

First Edition : **2006**

ISBN 81-8061-797-1

Typeset at   JPBMP typesetting unit
Printed at   Gopsons Papers Ltd., Noida

*Dedicated to
St. Mother Theresa*

Foreword

I am glad to write the Foreword to *Spirituality in Nursing* book. Spirituality is an essential dimension being viewed in health. I have seen many articles and writings regarding spirituality. But many a time, concept of spirituality is confused with religious concept.

This book clearly differentiates spirituality with religion and gives the correlation between spirituality and health. Since this book is focusing wholly on nurses' viewpoint, this will influence all levels of nursing students and nurses.

Here, author has clearly given the idea about spirituality. He guides nurses to apply spiritual dimension in nursing process. The simple language and terms make this concept understandable.

I really appreciate the author for taking effort to make this book simple and easy for nurses.

I hope that this book will be a better beginning for practicing spirituality in nursing in Indian context.

I wish the author all the best.

Mr Yadidya
Principal
Shekhar College of Nursing
(SMET) CK Palya Road
BG Main Road, Bangalore

Preface

As per World Health Organization's definition spirituality is also a major dimension to be viewed in health. Holistic Nursing focuses into all dimensions of human life. But the latest studies show that the most of nurses have negative attitude towards spirituality concept. Nurses strive to incorporate holistic care that includes spiritual care into their nursing practice. This may result from an inadequacy in nurse education that does not prepare nurses to provide spiritual care. I believe that this book will give them the idea about spirituality and the basic principles of spirituality in nursing.

My personal experience with professional people made me to write this book. Even professionals believe that discussion about spirituality is unwanted. I feel that this book will bring Renaissance in spirituality in nursing field.

AM Rajinikanth

Acknowledgements

I am greatly and sincerely indebted to God, the almighty for showering upon me his blessings to lead me safely. I submit my humble salutation to all my pioneers in nursing profession. I would like to greatly indebted to my parents, in-laws and my beloved wife to help me in all my writings. My sincere thanks to Principal, Vidyakirana Institute of Nursing Sciences for helping me to grow professionally and for his guidance in all the way. I wish to express my heartfelt thanks to Mrs and Mr Prof Dr Jeyaseelan Manickam Devadason, Principal and Dean of Annai JKK Sampoorani Ammal College of Nursing for their positive motivation and their support. I am grateful to all those helping hands and not mentioning of their name is purely unintentional.

Contents

1. Spirituality: An Overview — 1
2. Characteristics of Spirituality — 6
3. Lifespan Consideration — 10
4. Factors Affecting Spiritual Health — 15
5. Spiritual Beliefs and Health — 20
6. Assessing Spiritual Health — 25
7. Nursing Diagnosis in Spiritual Care — 33
8. Outcome Identification and Planning in Spiritual Care — 38
9. Implementation of Spiritual Care — 41
10. Evaluation of Spiritual Care Plan — 50
11. Sample Nursing Care Plan — 52
12. ASSET: A Model for Actioning Spirituality and Spiritual Care Education and Training in Nursing — 54

Index — 63

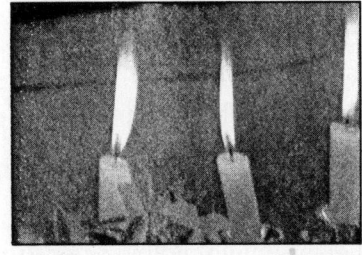

1
Spirituality: An Overview

"To remain well, individuals must stay in harmony with themselves, their environment and their creator"
—Carol Locust

Spirituality is defined as connectedness with self, others, a life or God that allows people to experience, self-transcendence and find meaning in life. Spirituality helps people discover a purpose in life, understand the vicissitudes of life and develop their relations with God or a high power. Within the framework of spirituality a person discovers the truth about self, about the world and about the concepts such as love, compassion, wisdom, honesty, commitment, imagination, reverence, and morality. Often, spiritual behavior is expressed through sacrifice, self-discipline and spending time in activities that focus on the inner self or soul.

The word "spirituality" derives from the Latin word spiritus, which refers to breath or wind. The spirit gives life to, or animates, a person. It signifies whatever is at the center of all aspects of a person life. A person's health depends on a balance of physical, psychological, sociological, cultural and spiritual factors. Spirituality is often identified as the important factor that helps to achieve the balance needed to maintain health and well-being and to cope with illness.

Frequently spirituality becomes equated with religion and privacy of an individual's religious orientation. But spirituality is a much broader and more unifying concept than religion. Florence Nightingale described spirituality as the sense of presence higher than human, the divine intelligence that creates, sustains and organizes the universe, and an awareness of our inner connection with this higher reality.

Religion and nature are two vehicles that people use to connect themselves with God or a high power; however bonds to religious institutions, beliefs or dogma are not required to experience the spiritual sense of self. Faith, considered the formulation of spirituality, is a belief in something that a person cannot see. Spirituality is also a component of hope, and especially during chronic, serious or terminal illness, patients and their families often find comfort and emotional strength in their religious traditions or spiritual beliefs.

Recently, nurse researchers as well as pastoral care professionals, physicians, social workers, and others have proposed that spirituality has special importance as the integrating theme that unifies all aspects of an individual's health. It is a force intrinsic to human nature and is one of the deepest and most potent resources for healing.

Spirituality

Spirituality is a concept that is unique to each individual. Individual's definitions of their own Spirituality are influenced by their culture, life experiences, beliefs and ideas about life.

There are two important characteristics of spirituality about which most authors agree:
1. It is a unifying theme in people's lives
2. It is a state of being

Atheist search for meaning in life through their work and their relationships with other individuals. Because atheists feel they are alone, they sense a strong responsibility for themselves. They also tend to believe in a joint responsibility for others. In acting for themselves, they feel they should also act for all of mankind.

In case of agnostics, it is important for them to discover or find meaning in what they do or how they live. Since agnostics find no ultimate meaning for the way they are, they believe that we as people bring meaning to what we do.

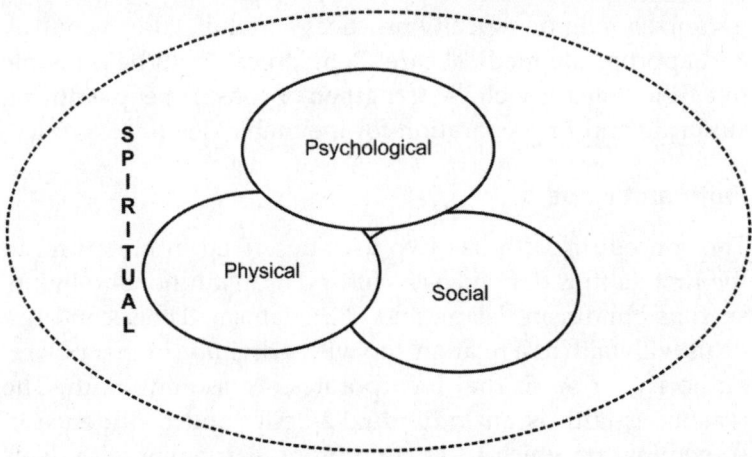

Fig. 1.1: The spiritual dimension: The unifying approach

Religion

Religion is commonly associated with the state of doing or a specific system of practices associated with a particular domination, sect, or form of worship. Religion is defined as a system of organized beliefs and worship that a person practices to outwardly express his or her spirituality. Many clients practice a faith or belief in the doctrines, and expressions of a specific religion or sect, such as protestant, catholic, orthodox, Jehovah's Witness, Judaism, Buddhism, Islam, and Hinduism. A person's religion influences the manner in which an individual exercises a faith of belief and action.

Religion serves different purposes in people's lives. For some, religion is a set of rules and rituals used to worship a supreme being. For others religion is a way of life providing nourishment and a connectedness to all of life. When providing spiritual care to clients it is important to understand the difference between religion and spirituality.

Religion often includes the formal organizational structures for social behavior. Religious beliefs can influence life style, attitudes, and feelings about life, pain and death. Some organized religions specify practices about diet, birth control, and appropriate medical care. Religion can both help people live fuller lives as well as strengthen or console people during suffering and in preparation for inevitable death.

Faith and Hope

The concept of faith has two uses described in literature. In the first, faith is defined as a cultural or institutional religion, such as Hinduism, Islam, and Christianity. The second use deals with faith as a relationship with a divinity, higher power, authority, or spirit that incorporates a reasoning faith. The reasoning faith is an individual's belief and confidence in something for which there is no proof. A trusting faith deals with the inner resources that allow an identity to act.

Spirituality is frequently identified as a key element in hope. Hope is described as a multidimensional concept consisting anticipation of a continued good, an improvement, or the lessening of something unpleasant.

Hope is future oriented. An individual imagines what is not yet seen. Hope usually includes active involvement by the individual. Involvement might include goal setting, caring, planning or praying. Hope comes from within a person and is related to trust. That which is hoped for is seen by the person as truly possible. Hope is more than a desire or wish. Hope relates to or involves other people or higher being. This can involve thoughts, feelings and actions that involve others. The outcome of hope is important to the individual. The expectation is often a future outcome that has meaning to the individual.

Hope is energizing, giving individuals a motivation to achieve and the resources to use toward that achievement. However, in either form, hope often offers new meaning to life, especially when a person conquers a disease or disability.

In times of illness, the thoughts of many people turn to spiritual things. The additional time to think, the uncertainty of life and the inability to control the course of events cause people to look for something secure and permanent in which to believe. Help is needed to face fears of death, past actions, life after death and to know what God is like. People want to know how to have a peaceful heart. They need to feel love and concern for their spiritual welfare.

Spirituality in Holistic Health Care

For nursing to be holistic, it should be universally applicable, cover all aspects of health, i.e. physical, mental, social and spiritual.

Ayurveda has a holistic concept of Medicare and health care and it defines health as svasthya. "to be one's own spiritual self". Charka (AD 500-600); the renowned Ayurveda physician, defined health as equipoise state of body, mind, sense organs and soul.

Swami Vivekananda said, "Serve every person as god." This concept alone can bring a revolutionary change in our attitudes in Medicare. This concept pleads with our health care team members to consider treatment of their patients as service of God himself. They would be making their profession itself a spiritual practice, through which great spiritual graces like peace, sympathy, love, freedom and fearlessness can flow.

Louis Pasteur, the great French scientist, said, "blessed is he who carries within himself God, an ideal beauty, for therein lie springs of great thought and great action." This brings us to the topic of harnessing spirituality in the scheme of holistic health care.

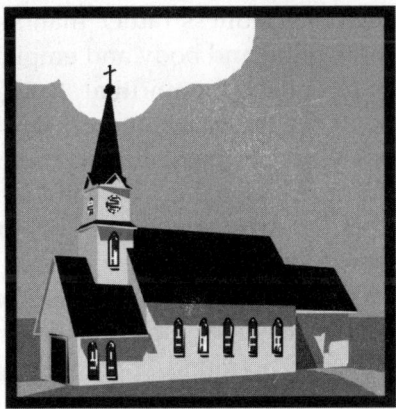

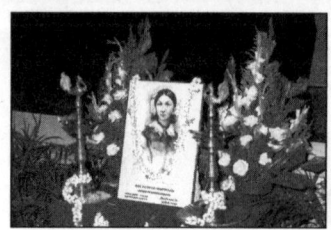

2
Characteristics of Spirituality

"The treatment of a part should not be attempted without treatment of the entirety"
—Plato

The major characteristics of spirituality include a sense of wholeness and harmony within one's self, with God or a higher power as one defines it. People, according to their developmental level, experience and project personal security, strong identity, and a sense of hope. It does not mean that individuals are totally satisfied with life or have all the answers. Assisting clients with the ensuring spiritual struggle is a valid and important aspect of maintaining health and giving health care.

Holism

Holism, the position of viewing the universe as a system of harmonious interconnectedness rather than sum of isolated parts, integrates the mind and body and emphasizes spirit. A holistic approach recognizes the spiritual struggle as valid and important aspects of health and health care. It is the integrating factor of" previously compartmentalized constructs of physical body, rational mind, emotional psyche, and intuitive spirit".

The concept of a spiritual wellness program has been introduced in some long-term care facilities. In this program, a spiritual wellness staff uses a holistic approach to care in order to address the needs of older residents, their family members, and the staff. Sigmund Freud's early disciple Carl Jung expanded the concept of the unconscious to make it include good emotions and even spiritual urges.

Spiritual Need

Definitions of spiritual need vary according to each author's belief system. In summarizing the various definitions, spiritual need represents a normal expression of a person's inner being that seeks meaning in all experience and a dynamic relationship with self, others and to the supreme other as the person defines it. Spiritual needs includes trust, forgiveness, love and relatedness, faith, creativity and hope, meaning and purpose and grace.

Spiritual needs are identified, as an individual's desire to find meaning and purpose in life, pain and death. The spiritual realms are often considered a very private area. In order to provide a holistic care, however, the nurse must pay attention to the spiritual dimension of each client, recognizing spiritual needs and assisting the client in meeting them.

Spiritual Quest

Life may be viewed as a spiritual quest, not only to answer life's philosophic questions but also to seek a higher level of consciousness or a deeper awareness of spiritual life. For example, the recovery as a spiritual journey; group members practice a spiritual discipline to live more meaningfully day-by-day. Recovery begins through a "leap of faith" which lays that there is no meaning to be found other than that which is beyond one's self. That which transcends man's ability to know that which is God.

A common question asked by spiritual seekers is, to what extent they should pay attention to their health. For some seekers this question arises because interest in spiritual life, which is primarily a quest for the eternal, immutable, ever-pure, immortal, infinite spirit, seems to be incompatible with interest in the ever changing, impure, limited, perishable physical body.

Spiritual Well-being

Spiritual wellness manifests as inner strength and peace. Spiritual well-being is a condition marked by an affirmation of life, peace, harmony, and a sense of interconnectedness with God, self, community and environment that nurtures and celebrates wholeness. In the hierarchy of human needs, spiritual well-being appears to connote fulfillment of needs beyond the self actualization level. All the subjects expressed a belief in a supreme being, had some means of communication with that entity through prayer and worship, and had an extensive social support system of meaningful personal relationships.

Dossey and Dossey(1998) state that the richness of a person's interactions with others correlates with positive health outcomes, and that practice of any religion correlates with greater health and increased longevity.

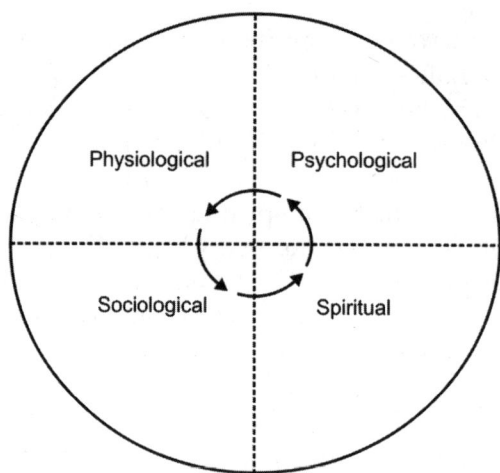

Fig. 2.1: Spiritual dimension: Integrated approach

Nurses are not asked to take over the role of spiritual counselors. Rather, nurses are encouraged to integrate a holistic approach by extending love, compassion and empathy;

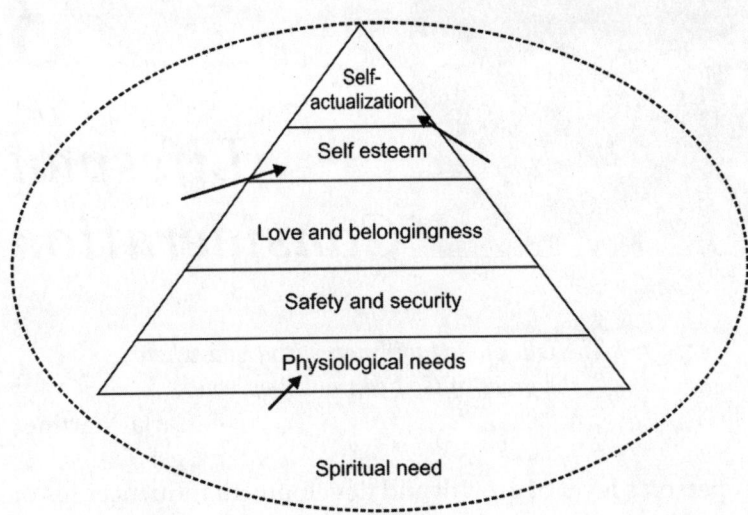

Fig. 2.2: Spiritual need: Maslow's dimension

motivating clients to address the spiritual issues; and suggesting how they might do so.

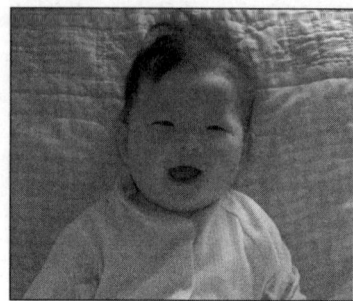

3
Lifespan Consideration

> *" The will of God will never lead you where
> the grace of God can not keep you"*
> —Carla Martinez

A person's level of growth and development influences his or her spiritual expression. Building on the theories of Erickson and Piaget, Fowler (1981) formulated a theory of faith development as the person's integrating center of valuing. Fowler's theory does not address the content of a person's faith such as a specific religious belief system, but views faith as another way of knowing the world, a spiritual knowing based on a particular phase of psychological and cognitive development.

The following explanation integrates faith stage concepts with growth and development and identifies spiritual needs arising from these stages.

Newborn and Infant

Trust in caregivers is the basis not only for development of a sense of safety, security of self in the world, and interpersonal relationship but also for faith development. Human beings' initial knowledge of the world is through relationship. If parents who are secure and have a sense of meaning and commitment meet basic trust needs, infants will sense this kinesthically and incorporate this feeling into their "inner most being".

Toddler and Preschooler

The first stage of faith development, intuitive-projective, is characterized by a continuing differentiation of self from others

Table 3.1: Fowler's stage of faith

Stage	Age	Characteristic
Pre stage: Undifferentiated Faith	Infant	Trust, hope and love complete with environmental inconsistencies or threats of abandonment
Stage 1: Intuitive-projective Faith	Toddler and preschooler	Imitates parental behaviors and attitudes about religion and spirituality. Has no real understanding of spiritual concepts
Stage 2: Mythical-literal faith	School-age child	Accepts existence of a deity. Religious and moral beliefs are symbolized by stories. Appreciate others view point. Accept concept of reciprocal fairness
Stage 3: Synthetic-conventional faith	Adolescent	Questions values and religious beliefs in an attempt to form own identity
Stage 4: Individuative-reflective faith	Late adolescent and young adult	Assumes responsibility for own attitudes and beliefs
Stage 5: Conjunctive faith	Adult	Integrates other perspectives about faith into own definition of truth
Stage 6: Universalizing faith	Adult	Makes concept of love and justice tangible

and an awakening of consciousness and memory. The introduction of language and gestures facilitates the child's ability to participate in some faith rituals of family's religion. Children will respond to routines such as grace before meals, bedtime stories and prayers, special celebration, and holidays if they are offered as a consistent, natural part of family life. Children also respond positively to those who treat seriously their questions about the world, life and death. Though children do not know about such matters rationally, they intuitively sense the deeper spiritual questions of existence.

School Age Child and Adolescent

Children notice the difference between themselves as individuals and others in similar or different groups. They continue to be sensitive to good-bad issues, often trying to "make up" for wrong doing in concrete, literal ways.

Children can now think in a historical perspective and see themselves as part of their family tree. The use of "story" is a major strategy for giving meaning to experience. Childhood is the period when the lore, legends, language and symbols of a particular religious group are best presented. Wishes, needs, facts and fantasy may appear somewhat confused, but children are attempting to make sense of the world. This period is the mythic-literal period.

The major change in adolescence is the beginning of the ability to think abstractly, to conceptualize, and to synthesize. Adolescents can ask more sophisticated, philosophic questions, test the truth, evaluate others behavior, and note incongruities. They develop their own personal style, based on their beliefs, attitudes and values. Although adolescents they carry out this function mainly within the peer group. Mutuality and interpersonal relationships have major effects, making the development process both individualistic and conventional. Although the spiritual need is the same, faith is now centered within the peer group, synthesized differently from the parents. Authority has moved from the parents to the peer group. Thus the name for this stage is synthetic-conventional.

Adult and Older Adult

In the individuative-reflective stage, young adults move away from the conforming peer group and clarify boundaries of self hood and commitment. An encounter with people or groups other than those that provided support in the previous stage often precipitates this shift. Values, beliefs and attitudes change as a result of interacting in more diverse, pluralistic settings, which can be stressful and frightening. Some situations precipitating this shift include new jobs, international travel, advanced study or education, or new religious affiliations possibly intertwined with achieving intimate relationships, choosing careers and starting families. The challenge during this stage is to establish one's own sense of faith and commitment based on personal experience and reflection on meaning in life.

The middle years are fulfilled through productive activity in Erickson's term, generativity. This time is of growth and renewed questioning, in some ways very similar to adolescence. Adults, however, deal with a broader world view rather than with group conformity. Older adults notice the polarities or extremes in life such as young and old, rich and poor, masculine and feminine, war and peace, constructive and destructive, and self-awareness and self-denial. These tensions enhanced or precipitated by personal and environmental situations, demand integration and resolution. This is referred to as conjunctive faith.

Table 3.2: Comparison of developmental theories

Stages	Erickson	Piaget	Fowler
Infancy (0-1.5)	Trust (hope) Autonomy (will)	Sensorimotor	Undifferentiated Primal
Early childhood (2-6)	Initiative (Purpose)	Intuitive/ Preoperational	Intuitive-Projective
Childhood (7-12)	Industry (Competence)	Concrete Operational	Mythic-literal
Adolescence (13-21)	Identity (Fidelity)	Formal Operational	Synthetic - Conventional
Young adulthood (22-35)	Intimacy (love)	—	Individuative – Reflective
Adulthood (36-60)	Generativity (Care)	—	Conjunctive
Maturity (60-)	Integrity (Wisdom)	—	Universalizing

14 *Spirituality in Nursing*

Most people do not achieve the final stage of faith, universalizing. Usually only great leaders such as Mahatma Gandhi, Martine Luther King and Mother Teresa appear to have achieved this world view. Terms such as justice, love and compassion describe the goals of the person in the universalizing stage.

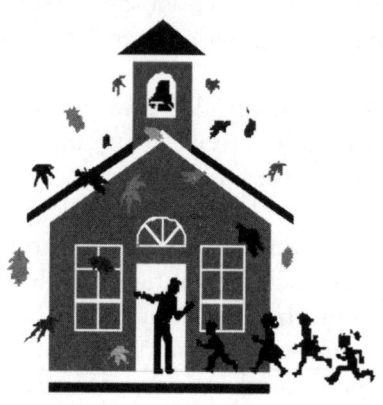

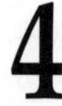

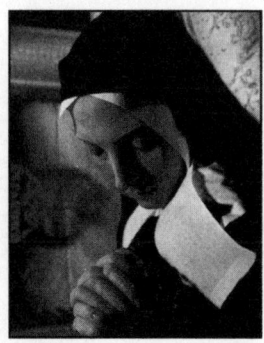

4

Factors Affecting Spiritual Health

"Look at the "ocean" and not at the "wave"…"
—Swami Vivekananda

A number of factor affect expression of spiritual needs. Such things include culture, gender and previous experience. Individual reactions vary depending on personality and past coping styles. Other factors contributing to spiritual health include appropriate religious education, a firm spiritual identity, a dynamic and adaptable belief system, and maintenance of belief system in times of adversity or under questioning by others, recognition of spiritual assistance when needed, empathy for other's beliefs and values, and a sense of spiritual fulfillment.

Other factors, such as crises, moral issues, and separation, can affect changes in spiritual health and well-being, placing individuals at risk for altered spiritual function. These factors, however, are subjective and mean different things to different people.

Religious Problems

Client's religious problems can affect their spirituality. Customary religious practices, if interrupted or changed, may affect the structure or support that religion contributes to the person's sense of well-being.

Change in Denominational Membership or Religious Conversion

Marrying a person with a different religious background or moving to a new community that does not have a branch of a particular religious group, will create, at least initially, loss for an individual. If a loss is felt, the individual experiences separation from a previously valued religious community. The extent of the loss is influenced by the choice the individual had in the change, how flexible the person's religious expression is, and what communities of faith are available to the individual.

Loss or Questioning of Faith

A person often finds a way to express his or her faith through religious practices. Persons who are at an early stage of development of their faith who find their faith challenged by an event such as acute or chronic illness, terminal disease, or loss of a loved one may become vulnerable to loss of or doubt about their faith. This can also occur when one is shunned by one's religious community or when one is seriously questions the position one's religious denomination takes on a public issue. A loss or questioning of faith can cause serious guilt and a sense of loneliness even when it can lead to more mature faith and stronger conviction.

Culture

Altitudes, beliefs and values arise from one's sociocultural background. Usually, but not always, people follow the spiritual and religious tradition of their families of origin. In inter faith marriages, children may follow the practices of one parent over the other. Many times, religious preference is tied to the ethic background.

Gender

Spiritual expression also depends on society's and the religious group's beliefs and teachings about gender or expected behaviors for males and females. A person's organized religion may prescribe how each sex dresses and if one wears a head covering. In same cases, the spiritual leader is always male.

Previous Experience

It would appear that if one's faith and values are confronted, then deeper spiritual needs would arise. During a crisis, past coping styles or learned ways of handling situations are likely to be evident. Life experiences in general are influences. Such experiences may or may not be related to age.

Crisis and Change

A crisis may strengthen a person's spirituality, which often happens when people face death. Just as crisis may strengthen one's faith, it may also weaken it. Crisis may be related to pathophysiologic changes, required treatments, or situations affecting the person.

Personal changes that result from the death or illness of a loved one, opposition to personal religious beliefs by significant others, or change in personal status can become other sources of spiritual distress. Being hospitalized can interrupt usual religious practices at a time when they are most needed, which can add to spiritual distress.

Separation from Spiritual Ties

Experience of being hospitalized or becoming a resident in a retirement or nursing home can initially be shattering. To some extent, such individuals are isolated from personal freedom, personal privileges, and social support systems. This separation from spiritual ties places people at risk for altered spiritual function.

Moral Issues Regarding Therapy

Many religions view healers and the healing process as evidence of God at work in the world. Certain groups, however, object to some modern medical interventions. For example, some Christians oppose abortion because of their belief that the soul enters the body at conception. Religious teachings influence attitudes toward many other medical procedures such as right-to-die decisions, organ transplantation, circumcision, birth control, sterilization, autopsies and handling of the diseased. The choice to treat may be difficult to make if the religious beliefs say "no" and the health care system says "yes". Many health care agencies have ethics committee to clarify and review such situation so more adequate and informed decisions are made.

Inadequate or Inappropriate Care

When dealing with spiritual care, nurses must be careful neither to avoid assisting clients with such care nor to involve themselves without desire on the client's part. Doing nothing

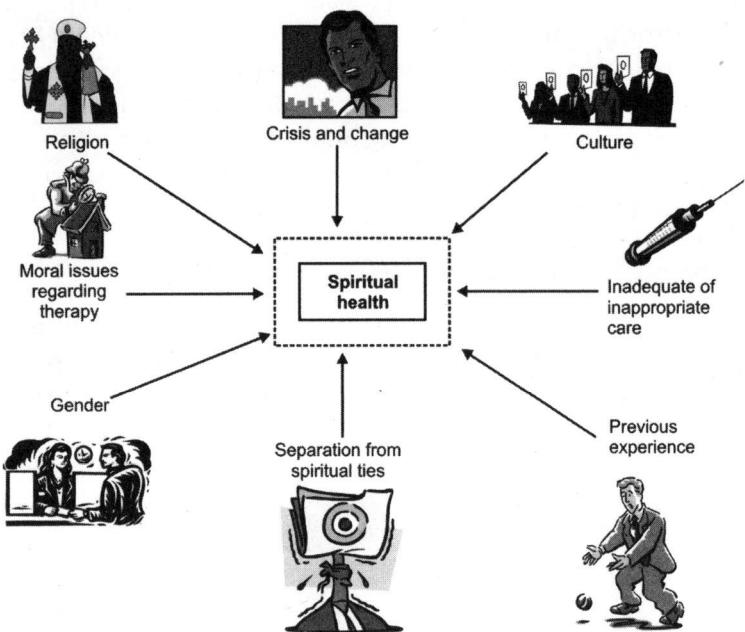

Fig. 4.1: Factors influencing spiritual health

or jumping in too quickly may result in inadequate or inappropriate care. Grandstorm (1985) elaborates on these reasons when she identifies five fairly complex values issues between nurses and clients.

Pleuralism: Nurses and clients embrace a wide spectrum of beliefs and creeds.

Fear: Related to not being able to handle situations, intruding on client's privacy, or becoming confused in one's own belief and value system.

Awareness of own spiritual quest: What gives meaning, purpose, hope and sense of love in one's own life.

Confusion: Confusion over difference between religious and spiritual concepts.

Basic attitudes: Attitudes relative to illness, aging and suffering. The nurses need opportunities to reflect on their own philosophies and belief systems.

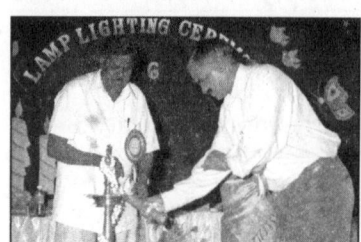

5
Spiritual Beliefs and Health

"To become a thoroughly good person is the best person is the best prescription for keeping a sound mind and a sound body"
—Francis Bowen

The Religious Support system is a group of ministers, priests, rabbis, nuns, mullahs, shamans or laypersons who are able to meet clients spiritual needs in the health care setting. The nurse has responsibility of working with these individuals, including them in the client care team.

Nurses must be aware of the general philosophies of their clients spiritual beliefs and also be aware that some individuals do not believe in a higher being or practice a specific religion.

The religion that provides satisfying answers to the deep question of the spirit and provides a worthy person to worship claims the devotion of the seeking person. We want religion that expressed love and gives courage in place of fear. Religions have practices relation to birth, death marriage and salvation.

Hinduism

It represents a 5000-year tradition. Its many different beliefs and practices depend on the culture and tribal unit. One medical tradition is the Ayurveda system in which illness are viewed as a state of balance. In this world-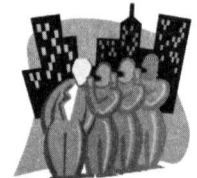
view, the human being is continuous with the environment. Hinduism has no common creeds or doctrines that bind Hindus together. The major distinguishing characteristic is the social

caste system. The religion of Hinduism is founded on the scripture called the Vedas. Brahma is the principal source of the universe and the center from which all things proceed and to which all things return.

Reincarnation is a central belief in Hindu thought. The goal of existence is freedom from the cycle of rebirth and death and entrance into what the Hindus, like the Buddhists, call Nirvana. Hindu temples are dwelling places for deities to which people bring offerings. Some Hindus believe in faith healing, others believe that illness is God's way of punishing a person for sins. In sickness they believe that the females to be examined by females. They accept modern medical science.

Their dietary rules are:

Wide range from complete vegetarian to restrictions on certain foods such as poultry and milk products. Traditional foods include many legumes, yogurt and spices. There is a belief system of hot and cold food, depending on how the body responds. Balancing tastes is also important. In some places, to refuse food means that one is angry or hurt.

At the death, some place the body on the floor or the earth to facilitate the soul's journey. Cremation is the common practice; fire purifies the body and the family gives the ashes to the holy waters.

Islam

The religion of Muslims is Islam. They believe that Allah is the supreme deity and that Mohammad, the founder of Islam, is the chief prophet. The Muslims' holy day of worship extends from sunset on Thursday to sunset on Friday. Some Muslims may desire to pray to their God Allah five times a day (after dawn, at noon, at mid afternoon, after sunset and at night). If the Client requests that he face Mecca, the holy city of Islam, a bed or chair may be positioned facing that direction. The Muslim client may be wearing an article of writing from the Koran on a piece of string around his neck, arm or waist. This should not be allowed to get wet or to be removed. Rules of cleanliness include eating with the right hand and cleansing self with the left hand after urinating or defecating. Medications or other materials should be handed to the Muslim client with right hand so as not to offend them, as they consider the left hand dirty.

Some Islamic females prefer to be clothed from head to ankle. During the physical examination, they may prefer to undress one body part at a time. They may refuse to be cared by male nurses or physicians. They may have a fatalistic view of health.

Pork and alcohol are forbidden for them. Islamic law permits contraception. Abortion is forbidden. Donation of body parts or organs is generally not allowed. Vigilant attitude is required to avoid misuse. They believe family should be with dying person so they can read the Koran and pray. Believe in special procedures for care of body after death; men wash male bodies and women wash female bodies and perform a variety of other rituals.

Buddhism

Buddhism began in the 6th century BC in North East India and expanded along trade routes to the South, South East Asia, China and Japan and in the latter 19th Century to the West. The medical system used is the Ayurveda system. The path of health is right living and thinking. There are many different Buddhist groups who follow different leaders.

Buddhism is a general term that indicates a belief in Buddha, "the enlightened one". Nirvana, a state of greater inner freedom and spontaneity, is the goal of existence. When one achieves Nirvana, the mind has supreme peace, purity and strength. Buddhism does not dictate any specific practices or sacraments. There are no religious restrictions for therapy or special holydays Buddhists do not believe in healing through faith. The religious support system for the sick is the priest. The Buddhist believes in reincarnation. They believe that nonhuman spirits invading the body cause illness.

Diet is an issue of balance, similar to Hindu beliefs. Alcohol and other drugs are forbidden because they can lead to moral

Spiritual Beliefs and Health

Carelessness. There is ambiguity about when life begins so there is no clear-cut view on abortion. They are against killing injuring humans and animals. Both birth control and abortion have been known and practiced. At present, there is no stated view about organ transplants. Prayers are said at certain times and up to 1 year after death then every year.

Christianity

Christianity accepts modern medical science. It uses prayer and faith healing. Appreciates visits from clergy. Some will use laying on of hands. Holy communion is commonly used.

There are many subdivisions and forms are there. They are:

Protestants

- Baptist
- Episcopal
- Lutheran
- Methodist
- Presbyterian
- Seventh day Adventist

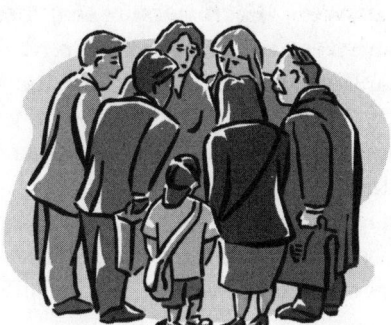

Roman Catholic

- Orthodox
- Jehovah's witness
- Mormon (Church of Jesus Christ of the Later Day saints)

Christian Science

The principles are same for all divisions but way of practicing is varying.

Judaism

Judaism is both a religious faith and an ethnic identity. The religion is based on the five books of Moses called the Torah. Culture and religion are deeply interwoven in the Jewish faith.

There are 3 groups in Judaism: Orthodox, Conservative and Reformed.

The rabbi is the spiritual leader of the Jewish Congregation. Circumcision is a religious custom in Judaism that is performed on the male infant eight days after birth. It may be done by the pediatrician or by the Mohel who may be a rabbi.

Judaism believes in the sanctity of life. God and medicine must have a balance. Observance of Sabbath is important and it begins at sunset on Friday and ends at sunset on Saturday. Euthanasia is forbidden. They require special procedure for care of the body after death.

Religions have systems of beliefs established to answer the questions of man's spirit. Religions do not all give the same answers. Each person searches for the religion that gives answers that satisfy his spirit. The purpose of religion is to answer questions regarding the spirit and meet spiritual needs.

Religious faith is often a very positive influence in the recovery of a patient. The person who has faith in the goodness, love and power of God and is at peace with God, with other and with himself recovers from illness in less time and with less complications. There is less stress in the person with a positive faith, which permits all of the body's resources to fight the illness.

6
Assessing Spiritual Health

"Together joy and sorrow come and when one sits alone with you on your board, remember that the other is asleep upon bed".
—Kahlil Gibran

Trust is strengthened when the caregiver acknowledges and supports the client's spiritual well-being. The nurse must remove from the assessment and care plan any personal biases or misconceptions. Typically one of the questions usually asked on a client's admission form is the client's religion. Such question leaves little doubt that the accepted position is that of a "believer". It is important for nurses to sort out value judgments about other people's belief systems. As nurses, it becomes important to accept and acknowledge others beliefs and not spend work time trying to convert others to our personal beliefs.

The nurse must be willing to share and discover an other person's meaning and purpose in life, sickness and health. Another important aspect of spiritual care is recognizing that a client does not have to have a spiritual problem. Supporting and recognizing the positive side of a client's spirituality will go a long way toward delivering effective, individualized nursing care.

Assessment

Stoll (1979) cautions that the timing of the spiritual assessment is important and that it should follow the psychosocial assessment. The nurse learns to consciously integrate an attitude of spiritual care into nursing process. The nurse who understands the overall approach to spiritual assessment can enter into thoughtful discussions with the client and gain a greater awareness of the personal resources an individual brings to a situation.

SUBJECTIVE DATA

Normal Pattern Identification

Several nurses have developed spiritual assessment tools. Stoll's (1979) guidelines for spiritual assessment are probably most widely recognized. It identifies four areas and suggests questions for each:
1. Concept of God or deity
2. Source of hope and strength
3. Religious practices and rituals
4. Relationships between spiritual beliefs and state of health.

Tools also have been modified for various populations. For example, Still (1984) uses different questions to assess children's spiritual needs. Shelly and Miller (1999) also developed an assessment tool, it is similar to Stoll's tool but some differences are made.

Model spiritual assessment tools are given:

EXAMPLE 1

A Spiritual Well-being Screening Tool

The JAREL spiritual well-being scale was developed to provide nurses and other health care professionals with a simple tool for assessing a client's spiritual well-being.

For the clients with the visual or literacy problems, the nurse can read the items and record the clients' response. Items on the tool comprise three key dimensions. Faith/belief, life/self-responsibility, and life satisfaction/self-actualization. If the clients score on any item, group of items or particular dimension is low; it may indicate an area to explore further.

JAREL Spiritual Well-being Scale
(Hungelmann J and et al)

Directions

Please circle the choice that best describes how much you agree with each statement.

Circle only one answer for each statement.

There is no right or wrong answer.

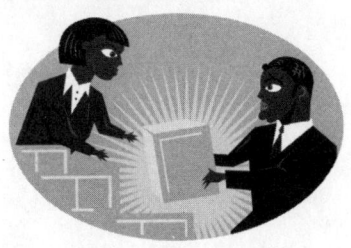

Table 6.1: JAREL assessment tool

S.No	Contents	Strongly Agree	Moderately Agree	Agree	Disagree	Moderately Disagree	Strongly Disagree
1.	Prayer is an important part of my life	SA	MA	A	D	MD	SD
2.	I believe I have spiritual well-being	SA	MA	A	D	MD	SD
3.	As I grow older, I find myself more tolerant of others beliefs	SA	MA	A	D	MD	SD
4.	I find meaning and purpose in my life	SA	MA	A	D	MD	SD
5.	I feel there is a close relationship between my spiritual beliefs and what I do	SA	MA	A	D	MD	SD
6.	I believe in an after life	SA	MA	A	D	MD	SD
7.	When I am sick I have less spiritual well-being	SA	MA	A	D	MD	SD

Contd...

Contd...

S.No	Contents	Strongly Agree	Moderately Agree	Agree	Disagree	Moderately Disagree	Strongly Disagree
8.	I believe in a supreme power	SA	MA	A	D	MD	SD
9.	I am able to receive and give love to others	SA	MA	A	D	MD	SD
10.	I am satisfied with my life	SA	MA	A	D	MD	SD
11.	I set goals for myself	SA	MA	A	D	MD	SD
12.	God has little meaning in my life	SA	MA	A	D	MD	SD
13.	I am satisfied with the way I am using abilities	SA	MA	A	D	MD	SD
14.	Prayer does not help me in making decisions	SA	MA	A	D	MD	SD
15.	I am able to appreciate differences in others	SA	MA	A	D	MD	SD
16.	I am pretty well put together	SA	MA	A	D	MD	SD
17.	I prefer that others make decisions for me	SA	MA	A	D	MD	SD
18.	I find it hard to forgive others	SA	MA	A	D	MD	SD
19.	I accept my life situations	SA	MA	A	D	MD	SD
20.	Belief in a supreme being has no part in my life	SA	MA	A	D	MD	SD
21.	I cannot accept change in my life	SA	MA	A	D	MD	SD

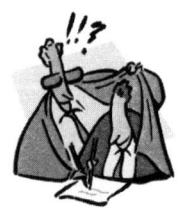

Example II

Davis M.C's Spiritual Assessment Tool

Client Name:_____ Date:_____
Days in Treatment:_____ Religious Preference:_____
Marital status:_____ Children:_____Age:_____

Part I : Spiritual Assessment Guide

In the beginning, share with the client that people have several personal aspects, such as physiologic, emotional, and spiritual and that this is an interview dealing with the spiritual needs. If the client appears to be very uncomfortable, clarify his or her concern and listen.
1. Spiritual ecology of childhood:
   a. Developmental history: Examples of some questions might be: Describe some early memories of how your family "kept" Sunday (or Saturday) or other Holydays. How did you feel about yourself? Your family? God? Eternity? Who taught about spiritual things? Can you remember any religions symbols, hymns, stories that had an impact on you? How did these experiences change, as you got older?
   b. Current religions practice: Do you participate in a religions organization? Do you pray, meditate or participate in same spiritual exercise?
2. Awareness of the spiritual: Client's awareness of some universal power greater than himself or herself and his or her experience of that power what do you think or feel about God? Is there an image or song that expresses how you feel?
3. Meaning and purpose: Client's concept of the direction that his or her life has taken, the present direction and who is responsible for life's direction. What meaning does your life have for you right now? When your feeling down or discouraged what gives life meaning?
4. Faith and trust: Client's ability to accept life's uncertainties and his or her willingness to trust and be trustworthy. How

do you view the changes in your life? If you were to get a box labeled "Your next major change", what would you do with it?
5. Forgiveness and grace: Clients' acceptance of others and self that allows him or her to confess and admit mistakes. What does the word "sin" mean to you?
6. Hope and creativity: Client's desire to make changes in life/life style. When you think of the future, how does it make you feel?
7. Love and relatedness: Clients' quality of relationships with family, friends, work associates, community, self and God. How would you describe your relationship with people?
8. Crises and peak experiences: Client's coping abilities and strengths. Have you ever had a time of crisis or suffering when you felt life no meaning? What happened to you during these times? Did you feel the same or different after these experiences? Did you try to get help from any idea or person? Was there a spiritual thought or expression that was helpful to you during this time? Have you ever had moments of great joy or break through? How has this affected you? Is there any spiritual image, music or art that expresses your experience?

Part II: Closing

Because this interview will stimulate a lot of thoughts and feelings, be sure to offer some clarification and summary time. Is there any thing we haven't discussed that you would like to add? Do you have any questions?

A nurse must be well in observing and recording in this assessment. Nurse must be aware about adaptive and maladaptive expressions of spiritual needs.

Risk Identification

In one sense, all clients suffering from ill health are at risk for spiritual distress. Even for those who have spiritual strengths, however, the time of illness and accompanying crises increase

Assessing Spiritual Health

anxiety. Certainly those clients with critical or terminal illnesses, who are facing death or other profound physical changes, faces ultimate, meaning in life questions.

Shelly and Miller (1999) identify nine situations indicate of a client at spiritual risk:
- One who is lonely and has few, if any visitors.
- One who expresses some apprehensions and fears?
- One whose illness may have some connection with his or her emotions or religions attitudes.
- One who is facing surgery?
- One whose surgery or illness forces him or her to change his or her way of living.
- One who seems to be doing more than the average amount of thinking about the relationship of his or her religion to his or her health?
- One whose pastor is unable to call on him or her or who has no Church application and so would receive no pastoral care.
- One whose illness has obvious social implications.
- One whose illness is terminal.

Dysfunction Identification

The discovery of actual spiritual distress depends on the nurse's observation of the client's verbal and non-verbal responses to the nursing history review. Identifying which spiritual need is lacking related to the nurse's ability to "listen with a third ear".

OBJECTIVE DATA

Sometimes in clients reluctant to verbalize such, issues, objective data are the only clues to a difficulty.

Glean as much information about clients from general appearance, facial expression, and eye contact, body posture and movement, sleeplessness, anxiety, and crying and inappropriate emotions.

Materials such as religious articles, books, cards and pictures also indicate the spiritual dimension, as do visitors from the church or clergy. Look for physical signs and symptoms of anxiety or distress that may provide additional evidence.

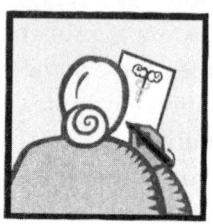

7
Nursing Diagnosis in Spiritual Care

"The Search for well-being is our human right"
—Chris Lovato

When reviewing a spiritual assessment to identify appropriate nursing diagnoses the nurse will have learned a great deal about whom the client is and the extent that spirituality plays in the client's day-to-day coping. As a nurse identifies the nursing diagnoses for a client, it is important to recognize the significance that spirituality has for all types of health problems. Pain, fear, anxiety and self care deficit are just some examples of common nursing diagnoses that will require the nurse to incorporate spiritual care principles.

Spiritual care diagnoses are addressed in the North American Nursing Diagnosis Association (NANDA, 2001) under the domain, life principle in Taxonomy II.

SPIRITUAL DISTRESS (DISTRESS OF THE HUMAN SPIRIT)

Definition

Spiritual distress is disruption in the life principle that pervades a person's entire being and that integrates and transcends one biologic and psychological nature. This may be related to practice spiritual rituals, a conflict between religious or spiritual beliefs and prescribed health regimens or a crisis of illness, suffering and death.

Defining Characteristics

The major defining and present characteristic is that the client is experiencing a disturbance in belief system nine minor defining characteristic may be present.
- Client questions credibility of belief system.
- Client demonstrates discouragement or despair.
- Client is unable to practice usual religious rituals.
- Client is ambivalent about beliefs.
- Client expresses no reason to live.
- Client's detachment from self and others.
- Client expresses concern and/or
- Clients request spiritual assistance for disturbance in belief system.

Related Factors

- Certain pathophysiologic, treatment related or situational factors may precipitate distress.
- High-risk, treatment related situations.
- Personal or environmental situations.
- Hospitals or others health care facilities may also present barriers such as ICU, confinement to bed or room, lack of privacy or lack of availability of special foods or diet.

READINESS FOR ENHANCED SPIRITUAL WELL-BEING

Definition

Spiritual well-being is the process of persons developing/ unfolding of mystery through harmonious interconnected that springs from inner strengths.

Defining Characteristics

The major defining characteristics are inner strengths unfolding mystery, and harmonious interconnectedness. A sense of peace, order and union with self, others, the environment, and God/ higher power describes harmonious interconnectedness.

Related Factors

NANDA has not yet established specific related factors.

RISK FOR SPIRITUAL DISTRESS

Definition

Risk for spiritual distress means that the person is at risk for an altered sense of harmonious connectedness with all of life and the universe in which dimension that transcend and empower the self may be disrupted.

Defining Characteristics

NANDA has yet to establish defining characteristic.

Related Factors

Related factors include:
- Energy-consuming anxiety
- Low self-esteem
- Mental or physical illness
- Blocks to self-love
- Poor relationships
- Physical or psychological stress
- Substance abuse
- Loss of loved one
- Natural disasters
- Situational losses
- Maturational losses
- Inability to forgive.

DECISIONAL CONFLICT (SPECIFY)

Definition

Decisional conflict is uncertainty about course of action to take when choice of competing actions involves risks, loss or challenge to personal life values.

Defining Characteristic

- Client verbalizes uncertainty about choices.
- Client verbalizes underside consequences or alternatives being considered.
- Client vacilitates between alternative choices.
- Client delays decision-making.
- Client verbalizes feeling of distress while attempting decision.
- Client focuses on self.
- Client has physical signs of distress or tension and
- Client questions personal values and beliefs while attempting to make decision.

Related Factors

- Support system deficit.
- Perceived threat to values system.
- Lack of experiences of interference with decision-making.
- Multiple of divergent sources of information.
- Lack of relevant information
- Unclear personal values and beliefs.

NON-COMPLIANCE (SPECIFY)

Definition

Non-compliance means that the behavior of person or caregiver fails to coincide with health promoting or therapeutic plan agreed on by the person and health care professional.

Defining Characteristic

- Behavior indicative of failure to adhere either by direct observation or statement of the patient or significant others.
- Evidence of the development of complications.
- Evidence of exacerbation of symptoms.
- Failure to keep appointments.
- Failure to progress.

- Objective test such as laboratory data that demonstrates improvement.

Related Factors

There are three categories of related factors:
- Health care plan.
- Individual factors.
- Health system and network.

Related Nursing Diagnoses

Possible diagnoses include:
- Anxiety.
- Ineffective denial.
- Dysfunctional grieving.
- Dysfunctional family process.
- Fatigue.
- Fear.
- Hopelessness.
- Impaired parenting.
- Disturbed personal identity.
- Powerlessness.
- Ineffective role performance.
- Self esteem.
- Disturbed sleep pattern and social isolation.

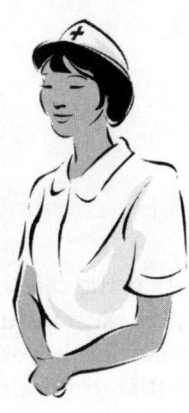

8

Outcome Identification and Planning in Spiritual Care

*"No creature can be sound so long as
the higher part in it is sickly"*

—Apollonius

As is the case in developing any plan of care, a spiritual care plan must include realistic and individualized goals along with relevant outcome. It is important for both nurse and client to collaborate closely in setting goals and choosing related interventions. Setting realistic goals will require the nurse to know the client well. In case where spiritual care requires helping clients adjust to loss of stressful life situations, goals may be long-term oriented. However, short-term outcomes can be established so that the client progressively reaches more spiritually healthy situations.

Goals need to be individualized by considering the client's history, areas of risk, evidence of dysfunction, and related objective data. Examples of goals for the client with or at risk for spiritual distress include the following.

- The client will express acceptance of current life situation including satisfaction with the meaning and purpose of illness, suffering and death.
- The client will participate in spiritual practices that are personally supportive and will express satisfaction with spiritual condition.

Outcome Identification and Planning in Spiritual Care

- The client will relate feelings of support in decision regarding health regimens.

Goals for enhancing spiritual well-being can be very similar to those for clients in spiritual distress. The focus is on supporting the client's strengths. The opportunity for spiritual growth may also be present as the client explores creative ways to deal with pain and sufferings.

During planning the nurse integrates the knowledge gathered from assessment and knowledge relating to resources and therapies available for spiritual care to develop an individualized plan of care. Confidence becomes as important critical thinking attitude as the nurse attempts to build a caring relationship with the client. Attempting to meet or support clients spiritual needs is not simple, and often the new nurse will require humility in recognizing that additional resources may be needed.

Caring must clearly be communicated between the nurse and client. The personal nature of spirituality requires the client to be able to speak openly with the nurse and to recognize the nurse's interest in his or her needs.

Significance others, such as spouses, siblings, parents and friends, need to be involved, as appropriate, to lend support. This means that the nurse learns from the assessment what individuals or groups have formed a relationship with the client. These individuals may become involved in all levels of nurse's plan.

In a hospital setting, one of the best resources to utilize in planning a clients spiritual care is the hospital's pastoral care department. These professionals should be part of the health care team, lending insight about how and when to best support clients and families.

If the client participates in a formal religion, members of the clergy or members of the church, temple, mosque or synagogue may need to be involved in the plan of care. Depending on the client's health status and needs part of the plan will involve a continuation of appropriate religious rituals.

The nurse must make sure that any icons or religious materials such as scriptures or a prayer book are made available.

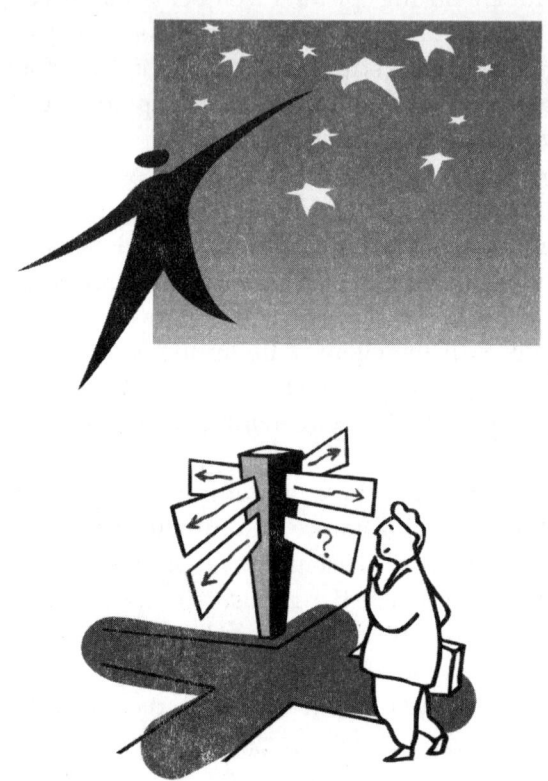

9

Implementation of Spiritual Care

"No attempt should be made to cure the body without treating the soul".

—Plato

Essential in implementing spiritual care are commitment to the nurse–client relationship, good communication skills, trust, empathy, self-awareness and acceptance of a broad definition of spirituality. Either the client and nurse must feel to let go and discover together the meaning illness or loss poses for client and the impact it has on the meaning and purpose of life. Achieving this level of understanding with a client enables the nurse to deliver care in a sensitive, creative and appropriate manner.

Although qualitative aspects play a large part in performing nursing interventions, implementation also includes continuing data collection; maintaining current documentation and collaborating with the health care team. Spiritual care is not limited to each individual nurse.

Health Promotion

Spiritual care can be defined as a mutual potential healing or integrating process in which the client's spiritual needs are met. Spiritual care should be a central there in promoting an individual's overall well-being. In settings where health promotion activities occur, clients are often in need of information, counseling and guidance to make the necessary choices to remain healthy.

Establishing Presence

Behaviors that establish the nurse's presence include giving attention, answering questions, listening and having a positive and encouraging (but realistic) attitude. The ability to establish presence is part of the art of the nursing. Presencing involves offering a closeness with the client, physically, psychologically and spiritually.

When health promotion is the focus of care, the nurse's presence becomes important in instilling confidence in client's abilities to take the steps necessary to remain healthy. The client who seeks health care may be fearful of experiencing an illness that would threaten loss of control and looks for someone to offer competent direction. The nurse's encouraging words of support and the nurse's calm and decisive approach establish a presence that builds trust and well-being.

The attitude nurse conveys when first interacting with a client sets the tone for all conversations. Listening to the meaning of what a client says is most important. It involves paying attention to the person's words, tone of voice and listening carefully to their story. By observing expressions and body language of the client, the nurse learns to find cues help assist the client exploring ways to achieve inner peace, take action, or do what ever a situation demands.

Use of Self

Spiritual care is a relationship that the nurse perceives as a valuable part of therapy and to which he or she holds a commitment. Qualities such as trust and empathy are partially built on good communication skills and an understanding of the processes and phases of nurse-client relationship. Without the establishment of trust and empathy in the relationship's first phase, nurses will be unable to discern deeper concerns such as meaning and purpose. Involvement in the meeting of spiritual need is very personal for both nurses and clients.

Supporting a Healing Relationship

A holistic view enables the nurse to establish a helping role. Within a helping role, nurse learns to establish healing relationships. Three steps are evident when a healing relationship develops between nurse and client.
1. Mobilizing hope for the nurse as well as for the client.
2. Finding an interpretation or understanding of the illness, pain, anxiety or other stressful emotion that is acceptable to the client.
3. Assisting the client to use social, emotional and spiritual resources.

Hope motivates people with strategies to face challenges in life. The nurse can help a client find things to hope for. Hope has both short and long-term implication. From a long-term perspective, hope gives individuals motivation to carry on with life's responsibilities. In the short-term view, hope offers an incentive for constructive copying with obstacles and for finding ways to realize the object of hope. To help clients achieve hope, the nurse and client work together to find an explanation of the situation that is acceptable to both. Then the nurse helps the client realistically exercise hope.

To further support a healing relationship the nurse must remain aware of the client's spiritual resources and needs. When the life stressors, or illness create confusion or uncertainty for the client, the nurse must recognize the possible effect this can have on a client's well-being.

Acute Care

Within acute care settings, clients experience multiple stressors that threaten to overwhelm their coping resources. The nurse works closely with the client and his or her support network in finding ways to make the client's spiritual resources becomes part of the therapeutic plan of care.

Support System

Support systems provide clients with the greatest sense of well-being during hospitalization. Support system serves as a human link connecting the clients, the nurse, and the client's life style before an illness. The nurse plans with the client and the client's support network to promote the interpersonal bonding that is needed for recovery.

When it is known that clients depends on the family and friends for support, the nurse encourages them to visit the client regularly. Encouraging the family to bring meaningful religious symbols to the client's beside can offer significant spiritual support.

Another important resource to clients is spiritual advisor and members of the clergy. The nurse shows respect for client's spiritual values and needs by willingly cooperating with others giving spiritual care and by facilitating the administration of sacraments, rites and rituals.

Providing privacy for the clients and clergy is a thoughtful and sensitive gesture. The nurse can help to meet the client's needs by careful, skilled and active listening.

Spiritual Support

Each client varies in respect to expression of spiritual needs and level or depth of spiritual case. Therefore sensitivity to this variability and offering appropriate care are necessary.

Nurses should not attempt to change faith that clients already possess. They should support and build on the client's faith. If faith is removed, clients will lose hope; without the will to live, many people are beyond the help of the most potent medical powers. The need is to make clients feel accepted in their beliefs and encourage to remain open in expressing and learning. Swami Vivekananda believed that spiritual ideas help cure diseases. He said," Even the poison of a snake is powerless if you can firmly deny it".

Diet Therapies

Food is also an important component of some religious observances. As with many aspects of a particular culture or religion, food and the rituals surrounding the preparation and serving of food can be important to a person's spirituality. In the event that a hospital or other health care agency cannot prepare food in the preferred way, the family may be asked to bring meals fitting into any dietary restriction posed by the client's condition.

Supporting Rituals

Personal care of the client should be planned to allow time for religious reading, spiritual visitations, or attendance at religious services. Family members can plan a prayer session or an organized reading of ascriptions on a regular basis. The nurse should be respectful of icons, medals, prayer rugs, or crosses that clients bring to a health setting to be sure they are not accidentally lost, damaged or misplaced.

There are many devotional and inspirational books and pamphlets that can be given to patients to read for encouragement and inspiration. Music and singing have a calming, comforting effect on most patients. Singing praise and devotional songs are effective in encouraging and lifting the spirit of patients.

Restorative and Continuing Care

For clients who are recovering from a long-term illness or disability or who suffer chronic or terminal diseases, spiritual care becomes especially important. Many of the nursing interventions applicable in health promotion and acute care apply to this level of health care as well.

Prayer

The act of prayer gives an individual the opportunity to renew personal faith and belief in a higher being in a specific, focused way that may be highly being ritualized and formal or quite spontaneous and informal. Prayer has been shown to be effective coping resources for physical as well as psychological symptoms. The nurse can be supporting of prayer by giving the client privacy if desired, learning if the client wishes to have the nurse participate, and by suggestion prayer when it is known to be a coping resources for the client. If prayer is not suitable for a client, an alternative may be read from a book selected by the client or from poetry or inspirational texts.

Meditation

Meditation can be a highly effective means for creating a relaxation response that reduces daily stress. When clients use meditation in conjunction with their spiritual beliefs, often they report an increased spirituality that is described as experiencing the presence of power, force, or energy, or what was perceived as God.

Supporting Grief Work

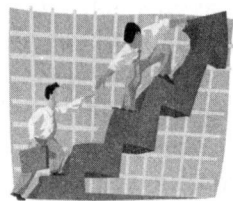

Clients who experienced terminal illness or who have suffered permanent loss in body functions because of a disabling diseases or an injury will require the nurses support in grieving over and coping with their loss. Supporting a client during times of grief can be strengthened by nurse's ability to enter into a spiritual relationship with the client, whereby nurse and client come to known one another as individuals. Nurses can prepare themselves to focus energy and set the stage for listening. Under extreme stressful conditions, some nurses believe in spirituality, themselves pray for the patients, which gives a psychological resilience to the sufferer.

Referral

If the client or family member asks for prayer or scripture reading and nurse is comfortable doing that, try to identify the special focus or topic before beginning. For effective referrals, nurses must have some familiarity with the available resources, particularly pastoral care, prayer, scripture, religious rituals, devotional articles, and sacred music.

Age-specific Interventions

Newborn and Infant

Hospitalization and illness potentially disrupt an infants basic trust in parents, the nurse can support the spiritual needs of parents by listening, offering support and promoting stability. Encourage parents to be present and involved in the caring process with infants as much as possible.

Toddler and Preschooler

Support families to carry out rituals of faith. If the family is unavailable to do this, nurses can carry out these rituals for them.

Young children are sensitive to good or bad issue. Do not tell them that painful or scary treatments are in any way a punishment.

School Age Child and Adolescent

Nurses continue to provide major support to families by carrying out familiar religious rituals in the health care setting. For children, classify fact and fantasy when it comes to all medical interventions and procedures. Acceptance and classification of the experience are the effective models to offer meaning to children.

For adolescents, development of a personal style and interaction with peers remain priorities even during illness. Involve the adolescent's peers by encouraging them to remain available either through visits, letter or telephone. Adolescents are capable of conceptualizing personal relationship with God. In times of illness, they may question the meaning of the experienced, trying to integrate into their lives, much as adults would do under similar circumstances. These issues can often be discerned during a nursing history and assessment.

Adult and Older Adult

Young adult's faith challenge is to establish and to reflect on personal faith and life's meaning. At the very least, all nurses must understand that young adults have the need for spiritual mentoring. Continue to be supportive of each client's family and social network because these relationships give meaning to the client's life.

During the middle year, adults become more concerned with a broader worldview and polarities. By accepting the possibility of mutuality in the relationship, the nurse has the opportunity to give new meaning and hope to the client.

As with other age groups, listening and support are essential as clients deal with health illness. Using a life review strategy, in which clients recollect past experiences and come to the understanding of them, is helpful. As infirmity increases, older adults may be less able than previous years to participate in their faith communities. At this point, facilitate connection with people or groups in the community who can either visit regularly or assist with transportation. Providing answers is not important. Rather the focus is giving clients the opportunity to discuss death and to make their own choices about how arrangement should be handled.

Special Population

There are differences in the spiritual concerns of persons with acute illness, persons living with pain, or persons facing surgery. For example, persons living with mental illness often have spiritual question because the mental illness can be in a form expressed in terms of religious delusion or hallucinations. Often, though, health care providers including nurses avoid spiritual issues for fear of "supporting" the symptoms of the mental illness.

There are new views of "recovery" as the spiritual need for hope. Hope is the "turning" point in a person's illness. So instead of avoiding spiritual care, several articles suggest way of incorporating into care.

Community-based Nursing

Assessing and planning for spiritual care comprise an ongoing process. Settings that encourage this process most consistently are usually those in which nurses and clients can establish relationships overtime. In acute care setting, nurses most certainly can become aware of client's spiritual needs, and begin to address them.

The follow up care can be more realistic. Some clients want nurses to prearrange visits from pastors, priests or other member of the religious community after their return home or transfer to another health care facility. Much healing and spiritual growth can occur without professional assistance because some clients find ways to meet their spiritual needs independently. Therefore, a sensitive and non-intrusive attitude on the nurse's part is crucial; nurses cannot force clients to deal with spiritual issue or to assume religious beliefs. Spiritual health is one area that cannot be put into a specific "road map" or trajectory.

As nurses we must turn our care more to the poor millions than to the well-to-do, who have another resources to help them. A sound health education of the masses would be the sure way to improve our national health. The last, but not least, would be to encourage the spirituality latent in everyone to assert itself, which can work wonders even in Medicare.

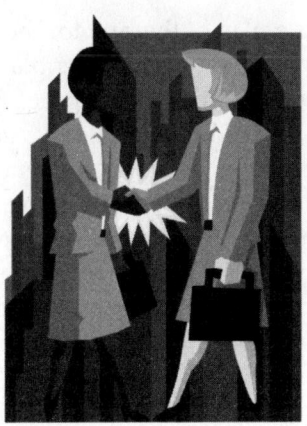

10

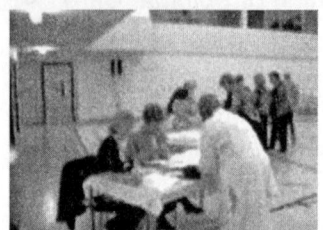

Evaluation of Spiritual Care Plan

"There is a balm in Gilead; to make the wounded whole.
There is a balm in Gilead; to heal the sin –sick world".
—Old Christian hymn.

Specific outcome criteria are the evaluative tools for measuring goal attainment for clients in spiritual distress. Outcome criteria need to be specifically tailored to each client so that the criteria will uniquely measure the client's attainment of goals.

The nurse will consider knowledge of spirituality and coping theory in evaluating whether the client has been able to adjust to those factors that threaten spiritual well-being. The nurse's evaluation includes a review of the client's response to care and whether the client's expectations were achieved.

Client Care

The nurse conducts a plan of therapy for the client's spirituality health while always evaluating whether planned outcomes and goals were achieved. The nurse compares the client's level of spiritual health with the behaviors and perceptions noted in the nursing assessment. Family and friends with whom the client seeks to have fellowship can be useful source of evaluative information. Successful outcomes should reveal developing an increased or restored sense of connectedness with family; maintaining, renewing, or reforming sense of purpose in life and for some, a confidence and trust in a supreme being or power.

For clients with a serious or terminal illness, evaluation focuses on the goal of helping the client retain faith and hope or expressing openly the uncertainties life poses. The nurse evaluates how the client is accepting his or her illness and whether hope has enabled the client to recognize individual mortality and focus on living for each day.

Client Expectations

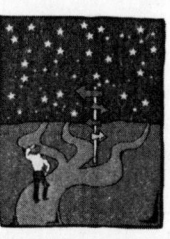

The nurse evaluates whether client expectations of the nurse and health care team were met. In regard to spiritual care, this involves evaluating if the client's spiritual practices were respected and if the nurse-client relationship was one of caring and supporting.

The evaluation of a client's spiritual care requires the nurse to apply critical thinking in determining if efforts at restoring or maintaining the clients spiritual health were successful.

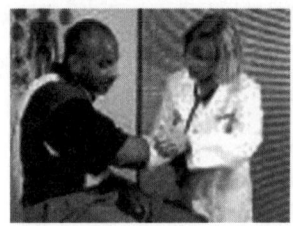

11
Sample Nursing Care Plan

Assessment

Mr Perianna, 28 years, who has recently been diagnosed with AIDS. During the talk and observation he expresses a fear of dying, anger with god, feels very lonely and difficulty finding ways to talk with his friends.

Nursing Diagnosis

Spiritual distress related to crisis of illness as evidenced by loss of meaning in life suicidal thoughts and over use of medication.

Client Goal

Client will express increased understanding and acceptance of current life situation.

Client Outcome Criteria

Client verbalizes feelings of despair, anger and fear after 3 weeks.

Clients identifies support provided by staff, family, and friends during periods of questioning and despair after 5 weeks.

Client identifies same alternative copying mechanisms other than requesting medications after 10 weeks.

Nursing Intervention

- Offer client opportunity for one on one nurse-client relationship. Actively listen to the client. Allow expression of negative feelings.

- Plan and coordinate a multi disciplinary team conference involving the social support network including family and friends.
- Explore past coping mechanisms including use of music scripture, prayer and relaxation techniques help client identify times when he or she can use a variety of these alternative strategies.
- Use the " life review " technique focusing on faith spiritual development. Help client explore ways to use this experience in a unique way such as sharing in a group or with medical students or other health care professional students.

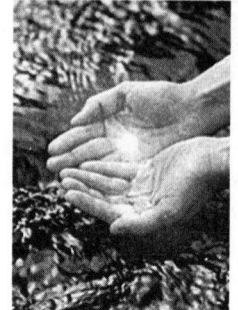

12

ASSET: A Model for Actioning Spirituality and Spiritual Care Education and Training in Nursing

INTRODUCTION

The model for spiritual care was developed by Aru Narayanaswamy. This model evolved as a response to the need for a clearer direction in the delivery of spiritual care education. Research studies in the UK and the USA consistently suggest that nurses knowledge and skills related to spiritual care are impoverished because of a poor role preparation in this area of care.

DEFINITIONS OF SPIRITUALITY

- The essence or life principle of person (Colliton 1981)
- A sacred journey (Mische1982)
- Giving meaning and purpose in life (Bradshaw 1994)

Spirituality can be defined as follows:

" Spirituality is rooted in an awareness and part of the biological make up of the higher species. Spirituality is therefore presents in individuals and it may manifest as inner and strength derived from perceived as relationship with a transcendent God. Ultimate reality, or whatever an individual values as supreme".

STUDIES ON SPIRITUALITY AND NURSE EDUCATION

Highfield and Carson (1983) found that despite the fact that nurse's learning opportunities include content about the client's physical and psychological needs is often omitted.

The need for nurses to increase their spiritual awareness is stressed by Clifford and Gruca (1987),They write: "Nurses need to start with self examination of their own spiritual values and attitudes".

Piles (1986) found in her survey that the fulfillment of the role of practicing professional registered nurses in providing spiritual care needed to be based on educational preparation for that role.

In a more recent study of nurse's awareness and educational preparation in meeting patient's spiritual needs, Narayanaswamy (1993) found nurses gave two reasons for being unable to give spiritual care. Firstly, Nurse education does not adequately prepare nurse to provide spiritual care. Secondly, spiritual care is seen as the realm of hospital chaplains/religious professionals.

In order to facilitate spiritual care education in nursing, the asset model (actioning spirituality and spiritual care in education and training model) is suggested as possible option.

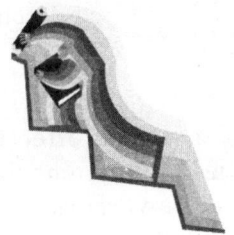

THE ASSET MODEL

The aim of this model here is to offer it as format for a stand-alone module or as curriculum themes of a course. This model can be implemented flexibly; however, it offers salient features related to the teaching and learning of spirituality.

Spirituality in Nursing

Table 12.1: ASSET model

Structure content	Process	Outcome
Self-awareness	Experiential learning related to: Value clarification Holism	Value clarification: Sensitivity and Tolerance
Spirituality	Perspectives of spirituality Broad aspects of spirituality	Knowledgeable practitioner in spiritual dimension of nursing
	Assessment	Competence in assessment of spiritual care needs planning spiritual needs
Spiritual dimensions of nursing	Planning	Planning spiritual needs based care
	Implementation	Competence in counseling positive nurse-patient relationship
	Evaluation	Competence in making judgment about effectiveness of spiritual dimensions of nursing Enhancing quality of care. Spiritual integrity: Healing and relief from spiritual pain

Self-awareness

Before nurses can instigate effective spiritual care, they need to examine their own level of spiritual awareness. It is widely acknowledged that training in self-awareness is a fundamental process before 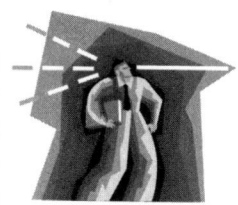 one understands others. Through self-awareness nurses could be helped to explore their own spiritual dimensions whereby they could be on their own beliefs and values, sources of hope and strength, meaning and purposes of nurse who has developed a positive attitude spiritual health is likely to be

sensitive to the problems a patient has concerning spiritual. In summary, self-awareness requires nurses to acknowledge their:
- Values, attitudes, prejudices, beliefs, assumptions and feelings.
- Personal motives and needs and the way which they are met.
- Degree of attention to others.
- Genuineness and investment of self, and how the above might have an effect on others.
- Intentional and unconscious use of self.

Spirituality

In the literature, spirituality is commonly explained from the following traditions:

Christian Theological Perspectives

In the Christian theological context an individual is seen as made up of a body and spirit. This is derived from anthropology of the book of Genesis when God breaths into Adam's nostrils to give him life.

More recently, the spiritual dimension of nursing from Christian theological tradition is explicit in Bradshaw's work. Bradshaw uses the Genesis account in the Bible (Genesis 1:27) to advance the theological basis of Christian understanding of spirituality. According to his account God created man and woman (humanity) in his image. Man and woman are unique and their nature is a unity, not a dualistic composition of physical body and spiritual soul as put forward by Descartes, but an entity in which the body finds expression in the whole.

In this respect, the significance of Christian theology is its emphasis on the "fruit of the spirit" and using this gift in caring for others. Paul spoke of the "fruit of the spirit", meaning those characteristics of love, joy, peace and so on, which the Holy spirit allows to grow Christian lives. Recently, under charismatic renewal movement, there has been a new awareness of what Paul said about the "gifts of the spirit" and the power of the spirit. Christians have looked for the spirit to give them love and the power of Jesus. In this respect, it could be assumed that these Christians who are engaged in caring may attempt to show something of Jesus greatness and humility in both word and deed.

In a way, it would be fair to say that Christian theology is responsible for reconciling scientific medicine and human composition, as a consequence of the refusal to recognize a distinction between spiritual and physical affliction.

Although writing from Christian theological tradition, Bradshaw has set the standard in her comprehensive treatment of spirituality in the caring context. No other work parallels that of Bradshaw's in the caring context presently. The position on Christian theological tradition, as advanced by Bradshaw, illustrates its connection and significance in nursing. However such a stance limits spirituality to being a specifically Christian phenomenon. It may lead to the misconception that spirituality is equated with Christianity, hence restricting reference to the spiritual dimension and its practicalities to the context of Christian patients.

Existential Influences

Contemporary existentialism, including those of theological existentialism emphasizes that spirituality is a universal phenomenon, in other words, all of us possess it.

The existential view is that we as individual have the capacity and freedom to reach towards our potentiality into roots of our beings. It is about those areas of human existence that are not accessible to the rational, esthetic and ethical areas such as truth, beauty, goodness, love, meaning and hope, which are the focus of human spirituality.

According to existentialists, turning one's faith or otherwise, as suggested by satre, Heidegger and Jung, spirituality is called into play.

According to Burnard(1988) atheism is the unequivocal denial of the possible existence of God. However, this does not mean that the unbeliever does not have spiritual needs or holds any sort of moral position. The unbeliever can be a moral person with a sense of responsibility for doing right and wrong.

Some humanists may relay on scientific reasoning and discussion to arrive at fact. Humanists also believe that it is the overall quality of life, which is important.

Agnostics, like atheists, still not discover or invest meaning in what they are and how they live. As argued earlier, the capacity for bringing meaning to what is within all of us.

In summary, existentialism illustrates spirituality as our inner potential motivates search for meaning and purpose. This view conflicts within conservative Christian theological perspective but opens up the possibility of considering spiritual needs of all patient's religious and non-religious.

It can be inferred from this that in illness it can be expected that every patient's need may manifest as spiritual needs and therefore require spiritual care. Indeed, the crisis brought on by illness might be the first opportunity a patient has to encounter the innermost spiritual being and, for some of them, the first opportunity to experience the meaning of their existence. Therefore, in the context of caring, Bevis (1978) asserts that existentialism has a great potential for nursing, in other word, the spiritual dimension of nursing as an existential phenomenon.

Existential analyses are used to provide many of nursing's current interpretations and understanding of the spiritual dimension of the human being and therefore reflect a more humanistic tradition, including the non-theistic, self-development and actualization.

Wright (1986) Writes

Models should be varied and dynamic things, which helps nurses in practice to explore and define their work, and should not confine them to a set order of being.

Steve Wright implies that when a nursing model is applied it may be in direct contravention of established laws, systems and social order. Wright's rejection of an imposed system or model as a basis for nursing practice is fully consistent with a radically existentialist approach whose fundamental emphasis is on spirituality as a universal phenomenon.

Although existentialism offers an explanation of spirituality that has a universal appeal it is lacking in the biological basis of spirituality as advanced by Hardy (1979) and Hay (1994). There is emerging evidence from research studies in support of Hardy's hypothesis that spiritual awareness is biologically natural. Any description of spirituality cannot be comprehensive enough without its biological root.

The Biological Basis of Spirituality

Emerging research suggests that spiritual awareness may be a human universal, hence in tune with the universalistic assumptions of the enlightment. The zoologist Alister Hardy's hypothesis is that religious awareness or spirituality is natural to the human species and evolved because it has biological survival value. Hay(1994) regards this to be more of a perceptual experience rather than a theoretical belief. Such experience, according to Hardy (1979), is natural.

As a note of interest, in developing his hypothesis, Hardy drew from the fields of psychology, animal behavior, psychic research and anthropology. Hardy's hypothesis led to further studies on spiritual awareness in many countries.

It will be noted that the 1987 British national survey suggests that almost half of the British adult population believe they have been spiritually or religiously aware, at least from time to time. In the light of other findings from in depth studies, Hay (1994) suggests that where there is the opportunity to build trust, this figure is boosted to about 2/3 of population.

Hay's qualitative research assists that people often experience an unity of spiritual awareness when they were going stress related to emotion, physical and or other forms of crisis. These experiences remain a personal secret because of the fear of others found out, they may become the root of ridicule, be considered stupid or even dead or waste. It is hoped that the current exposition biological roots of spirituality will open up debate in nursing.

SPIRITUAL DIMENSION OF NURSING

Spiritual dimension of nursing is the form of knowledge, attitude and skills from the above exposition on self-awareness and spirituality to nursing practice.

Practice

As guidance, an outline of the salient points related to the spiritual dimensions of the patient's needs is given for consideration when preparing nurses in the four stages of nursing process: assessment, planning, implementation, and evaluation an applied to spiritual care.

The Learning Process

Experiential and student centered learning could be used to develop nurse's communication and counseling skills. The teacher could act as facilitator to enable nurses to develop knowledge and awareness of patient's spirituality.

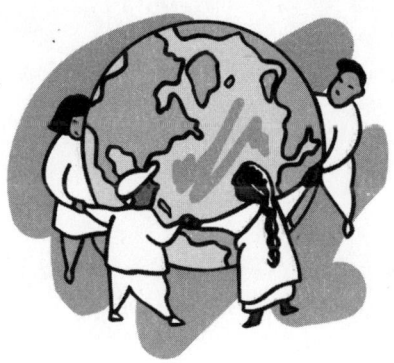

Index

Note: The letter *(t)* and *(f)* after page number in the index below denotes Table and Figure on that page

A

Adolescent 12
Adult 12
Agnostics 2
Atheist 2
Ayurveda 5

B

Basic attitudes 19
Buddhism 22

C

Charka 5
Christianity 23
Community-based nursing 49
Confusion 19
Crisis 17
Culture 16

D

Decisional conflict 35
Diet therapies 44

F

Faith 4
Fear 19
Florence Nightingale 1
Fowler's stage of faith 11(t)

G

Gender 16

H

Health promotion 41
Hinduism 20
Holism 6
Holistic health care 5
Hope 4

I

Inadequate or inappropriate care 18
Infant 10
Islam 21

J

JAREL spiritual well-being scale 27
Judaism 23

L

Learning process 61
Louis Pasteur 5

M

Maslow's dimension 9(f)
Meditation 46

N

Newborn 10

O

Older adult 12

P

Pleuralism 19
Prayer 45
Preschooler 10
Previous experience 17
Protestants 23

R

Referral 46
Religion 3
Religious conversion 16
Religious problems 15
Roman catholic 23

S

School age child 12
Self-awareness 56
Spiritual assessment 25
Spiritual behavior 1
Spiritual dimensions: Integrated approach 8(f)
Spiritual distress 33
Spiritual need 7
Spiritual quest 7
Spiritual support 44
Spiritual ties 17
Spiritual well-being 8
Spirituality 2
Spiritus 1
Supporting rituals 45
Swami Vivekananda 5

T

Toddler 10

READER SUGGESTIONS SHEET

Please help us to improve the quality of our publications by completing and returning this sheet to us.

Title/Author: **Spirituality in Nursing** *by* **AM Rajinikanth**

Your name and address:

Phone and Fax:

e-mail address:

How did you hear about this book? [please tick appropriate box (es)]

- [ ] Direct mail from publisher
- [ ] Conference
- [ ] Bookshop
- [ ] Book review
- [ ] Lecturer recommendation
- [ ] Friends
- [ ] Other (please specify)
- [ ] Website

Type of purchase: [ ] Direct purchase   [ ] Bookshop   [ ] Friends

Do you have any brief comments on the book?

Please return this sheet to the name and address given below.

JAYPEE BROTHERS
MEDICAL PUBLISHERS (P) LTD
EMCA House, 23/23B Ansari Road, Daryaganj
New Delhi 110 002, India